Special thanks:

(From the Author) To Martin, my knight in shining, and my two Topanga mountain girls Jensen and India... life with you is a fairytale! It takes a kingdom of support to write a book—many thanks to: The Ganz family; Mikayla, Dylan, and Jill Williams; Carrie Armstrong; Julie McInally; Star Oakland; Samantha Levy; Marilyn Levy; Donna Fedorowycz; Gala Calisto; and Dr. Craig Goldberg. Art designer Melissa Hertz, please take a long bow! Finally to Micah, thank you for the great magic of your talents. Encore!

(From the Illustrator) To my wife, Tiffany, for keeping me fed as I doodled away in my studio, my mom and dad for encouraging me to draw since I was very short, Luc Desmarchelier and Tony Siruno for the advice, and of course, Sue for creating this noble and witty story for me to illuminate.

First published by:
Wild Indigo
www.wildindigobooks.com
310-455-2400

Printed in the United States of America

Publisher's Cataloging-in-Publication Data

Ganz-Schmitt, Sue.
   The princess and the peanut : a royally allergic fairytale /
by Sue Ganz-Schmitt ; illustrated by Micah Chambers-
Goldberg.
   p. cm.
 ISBN: 978-0-9831487-0-8
 1. Food allergy in children—Juvenile fiction. 2.
Princesses—Fiction.   I. Chambers-Goldberg, Micah, ill.
II. Title.
PZ7.G1536 Pr 2011
[Fic]—dc22
                                        2011928329

The information in this book is intended to provide helpful and informative material on the subject addressed. It is not intended to replace professional medical advice. Any use of the information in this book is at the reader's discretion. The author and publisher specifically disclaim any and all liability arising directly or indirectly from the use or application of any information contained in the book. A health care professional should be consulted regarding your specific situation.

This book is a fictional work. Please do not attempt the acts described herein at home.

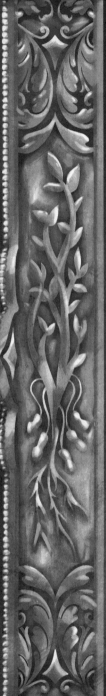

THE
PRINCESS AND THE PEANUT

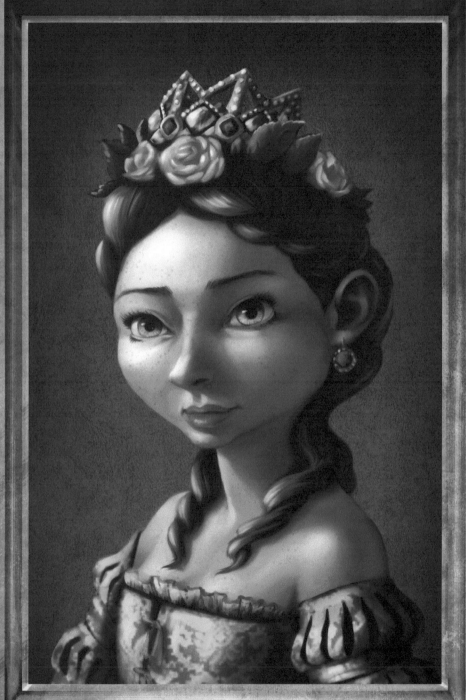

By Sue Ganz-Schmitt

Illustrated by Micah Chambers-Goldberg

Dedicated to Princess Olenka and her royal family

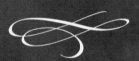

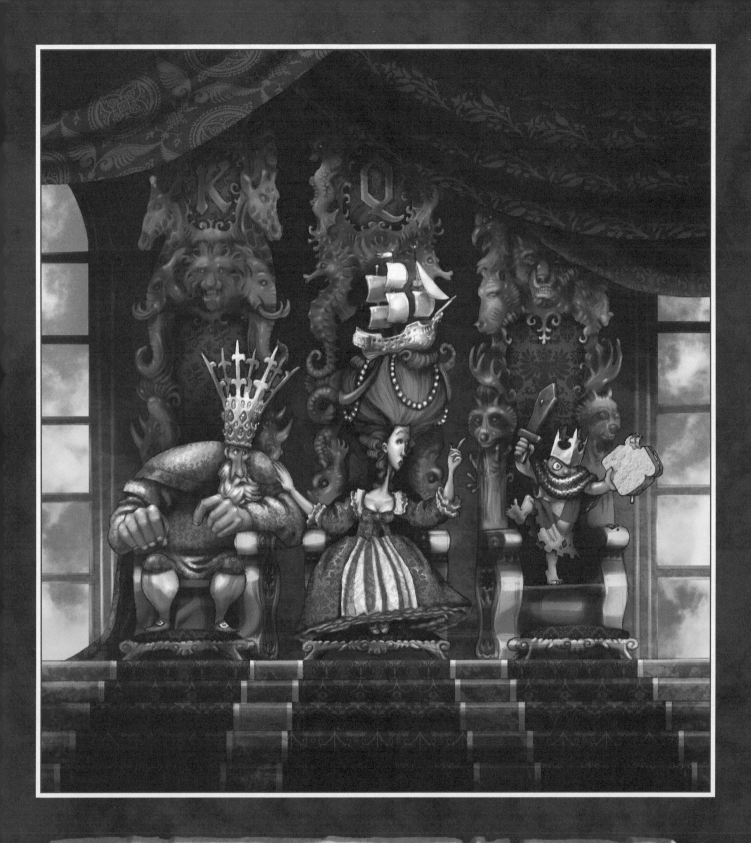

Once upon a long ago, in a kingdom well beyond your backyard, there lived a king, a queen, and a young prince.

When the prince was old enough, a tutor
was hired to teach him what he must know:

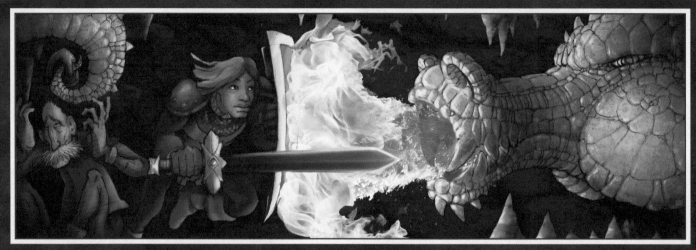

How to capture a dragon without getting burned;

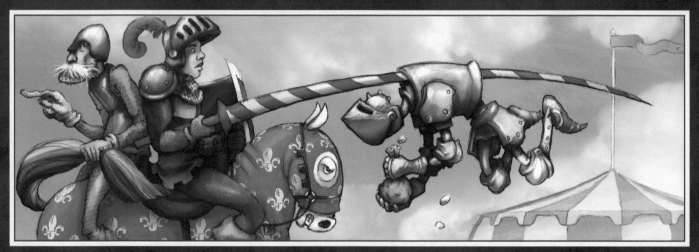

Jousting for fun and profit;

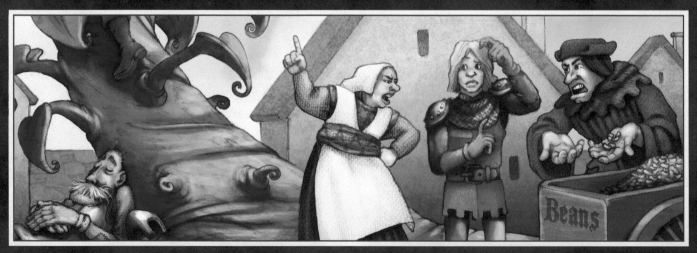

How to solve village squabbles;

And, of course, a prince must know...

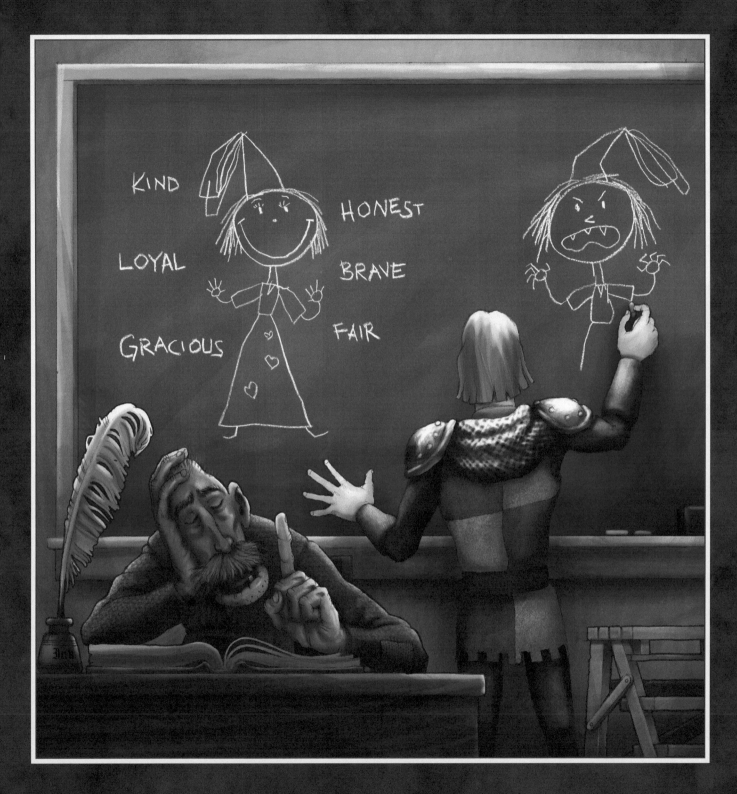

HOW TO SPOT A REAL PRINCESS.

When it was time, he set off to find his own, very real princess to marry. But it wasn't easy.

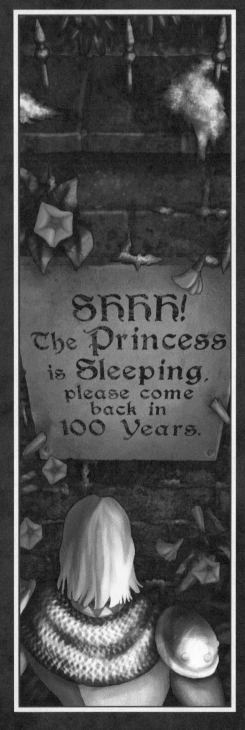

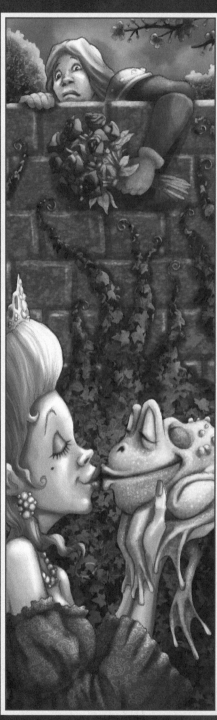

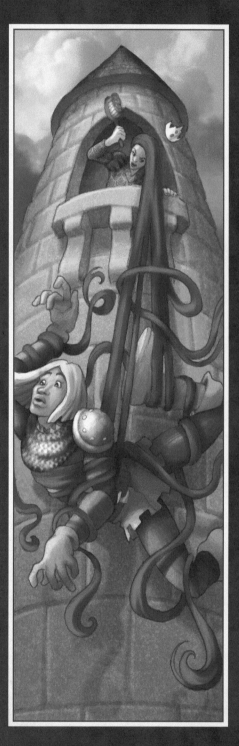

Some princesses were busy.

Some princesses were already taken.

And some were hard to get to.

Even worse...

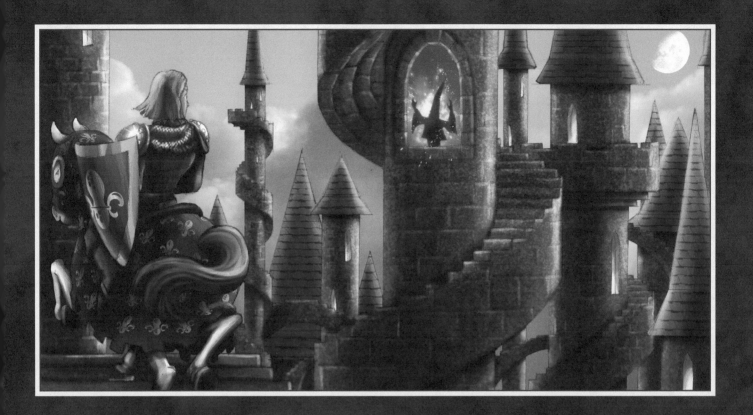

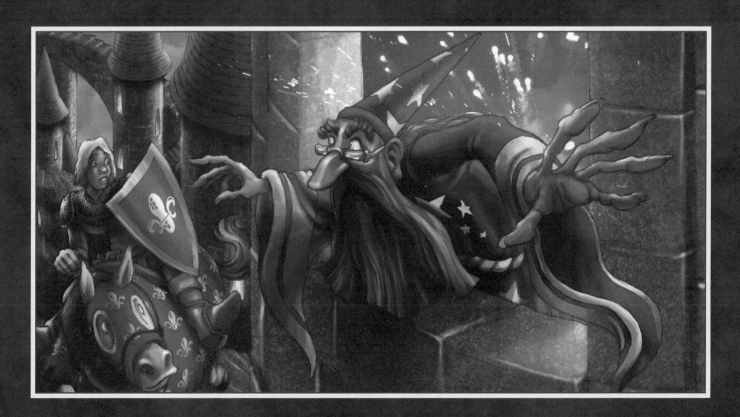

...some turned out not to be real at all.

Disappointed, the prince headed home.

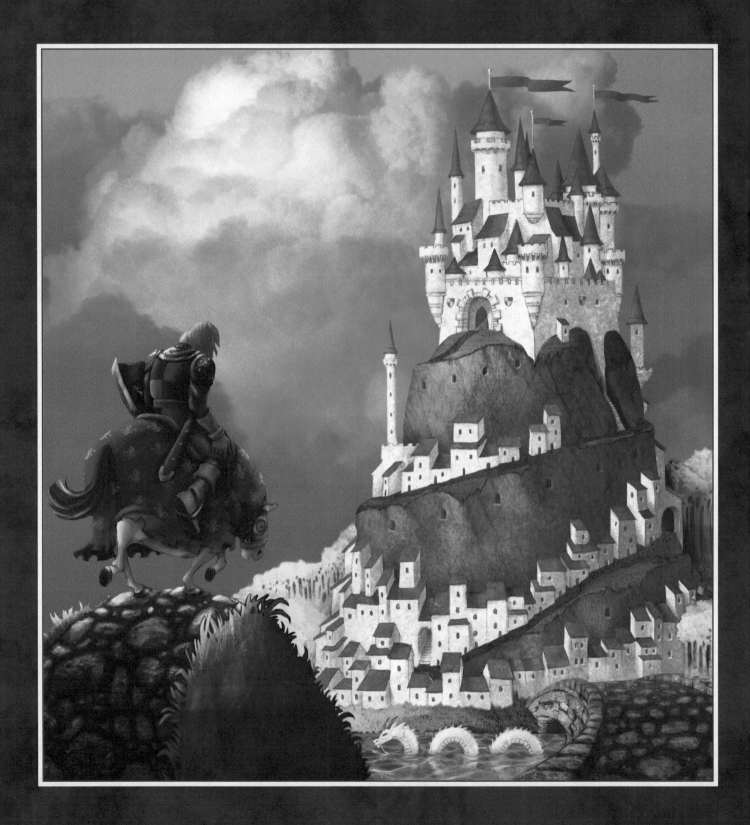

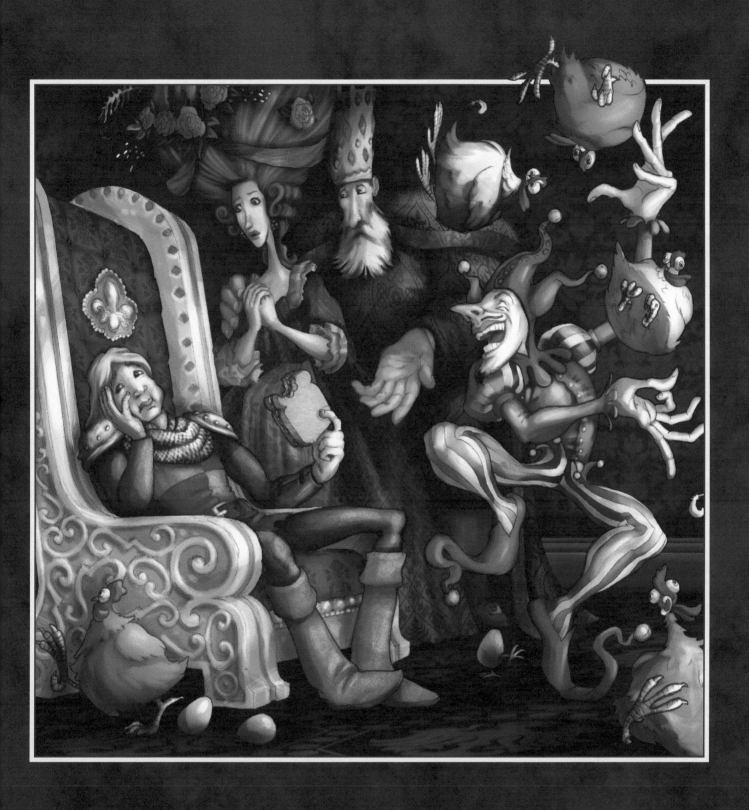

Neither peanut butter and jelly, nor the jester could cheer him up.

"I have searched the highlands...

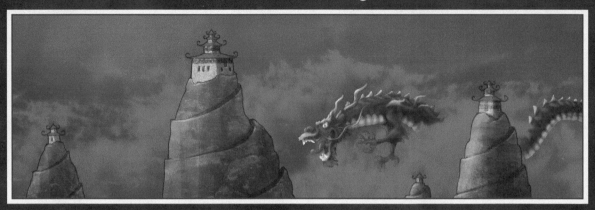

and the lowlands,

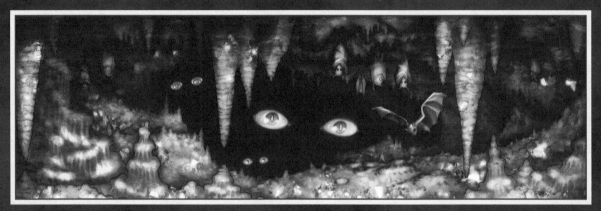

the widelands...

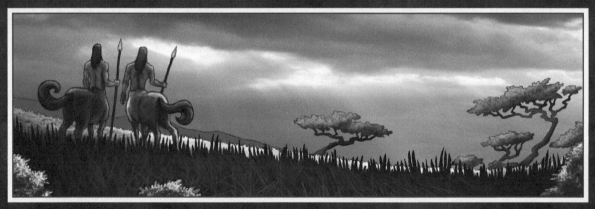

and the tidelands.

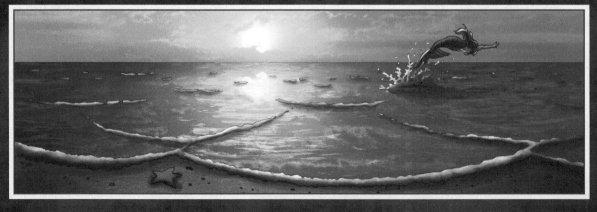

Perhaps I shall never find my real princess!" cried the prince.

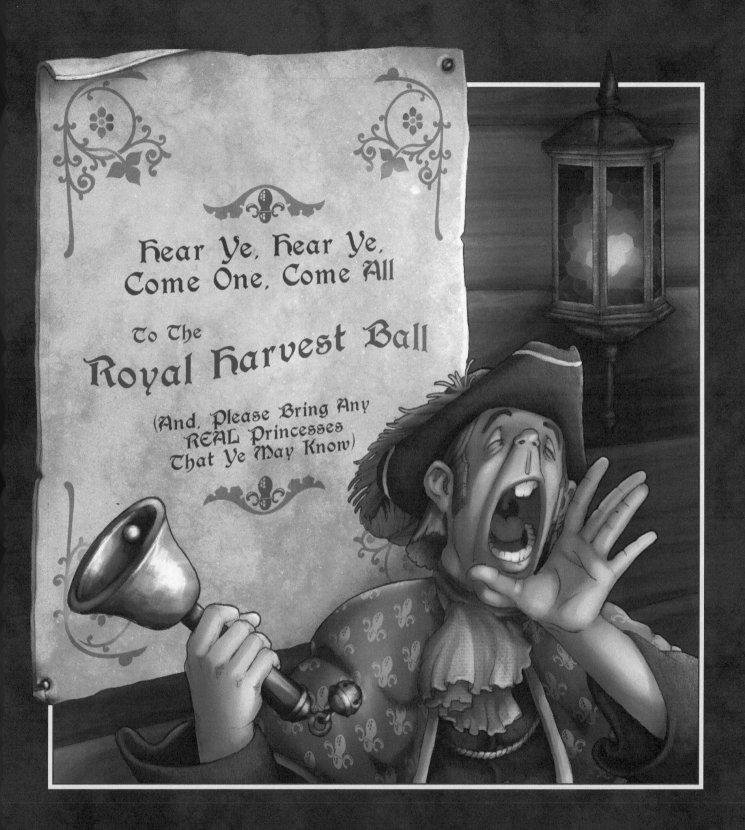

"Never say never," said the king.

"I know what to do!" exclaimed the queen.

Invitations were sent. And signs were posted.

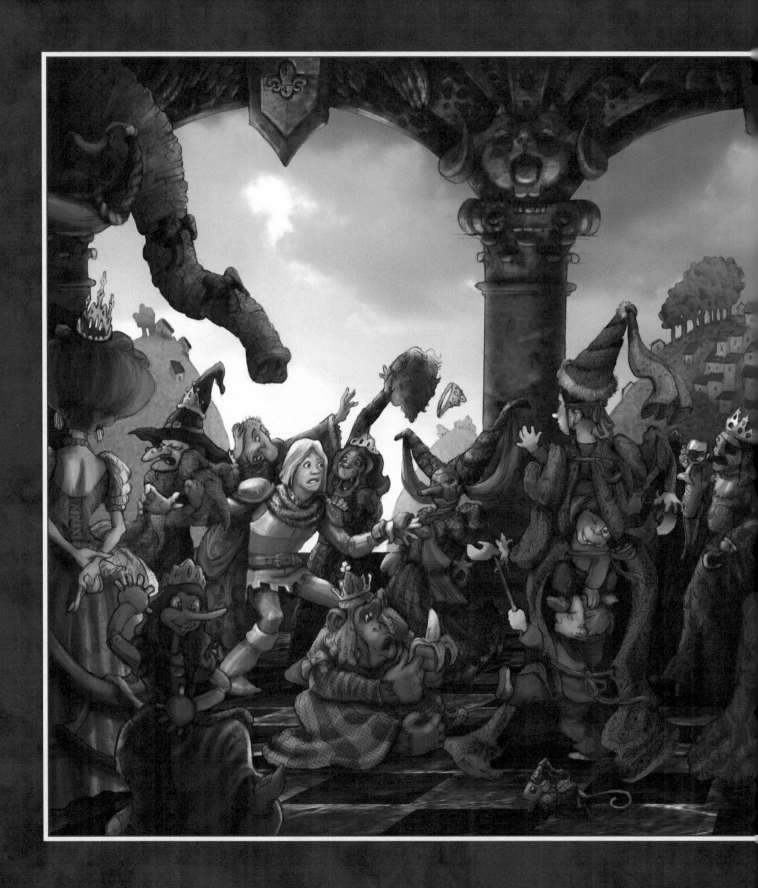

The guests were many. They ate and danced.

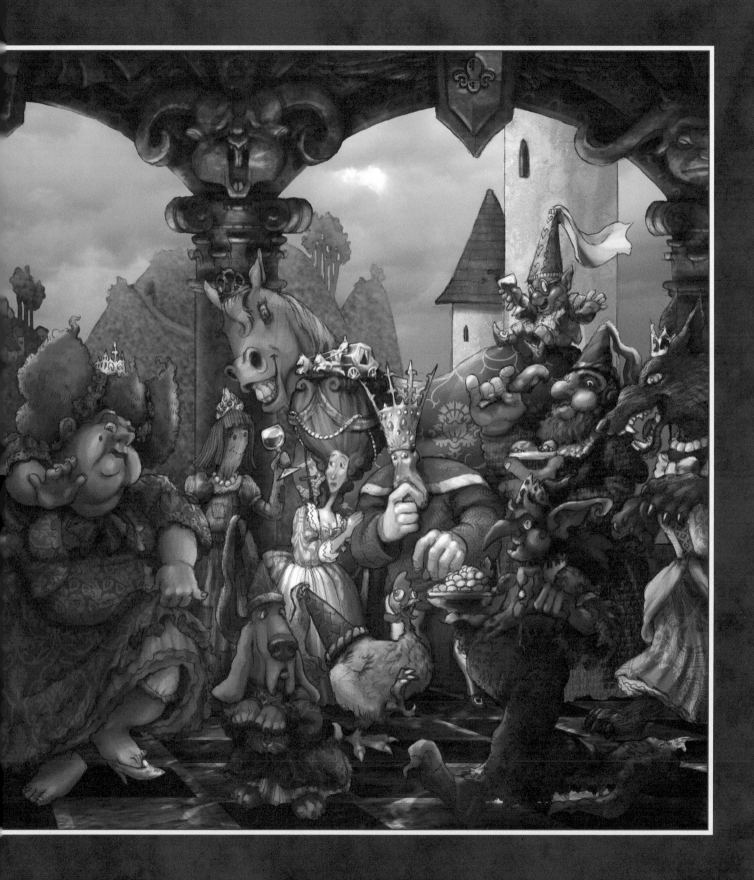

But there was not a real princess in sight!

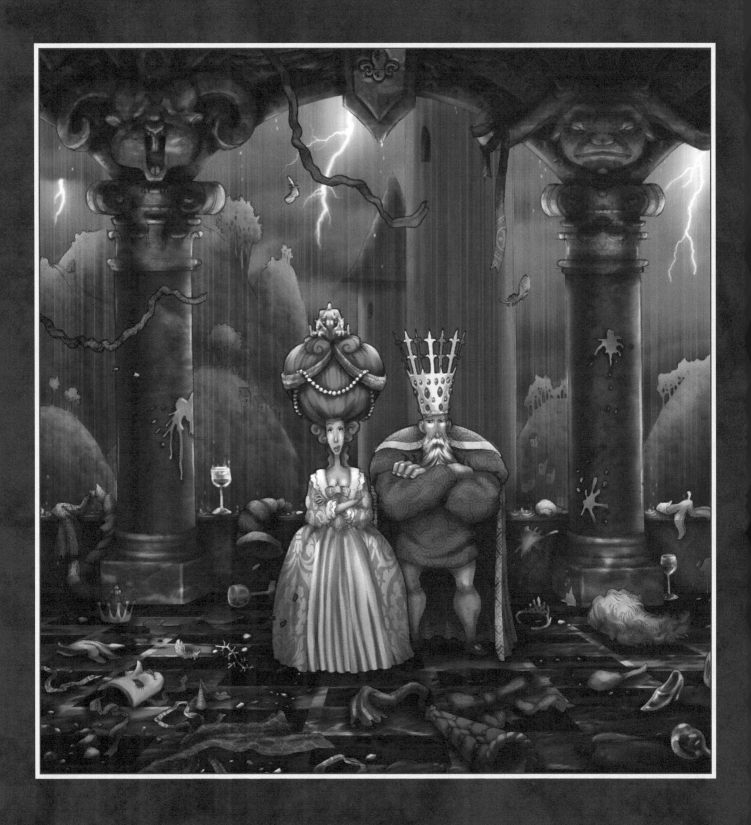

A royal sigh escaped the queen as the last guests trotted home. The castle gates were closed.

In a flash, thunder cracked the sky. Rain poured down.

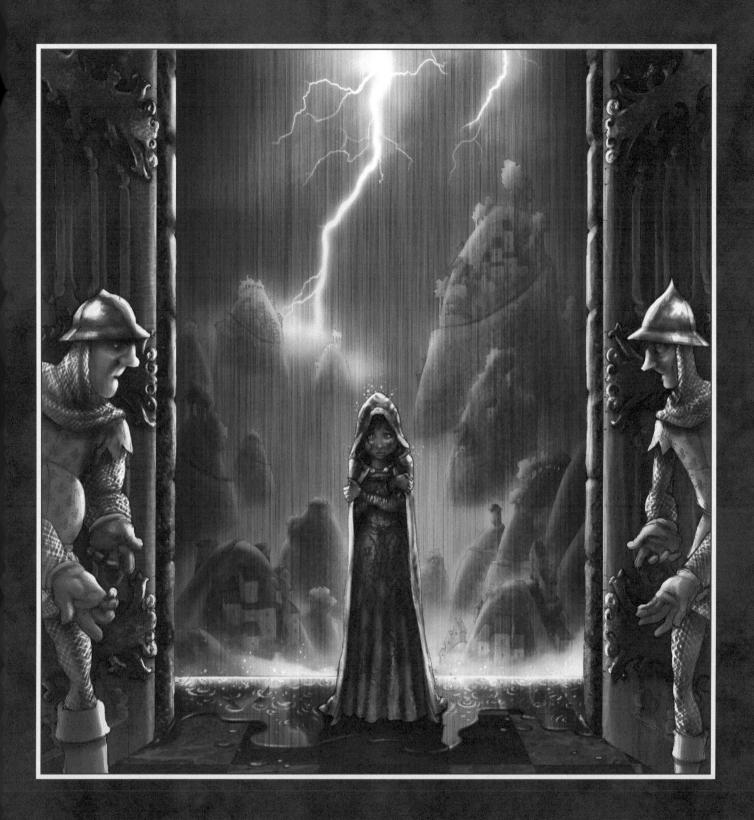

A bell clanged at the gate. And in the rain, at the gate, the castle guards found a maiden in tatters and muddy splatters.

"Do pardon me! I am royally lost!" said the maiden, and told her story.

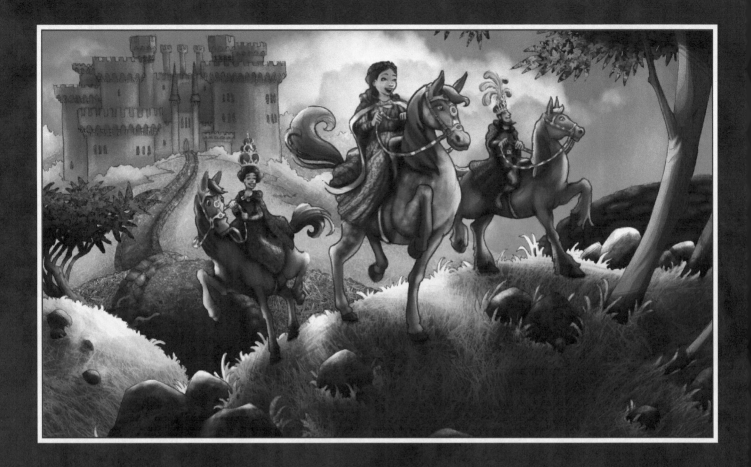

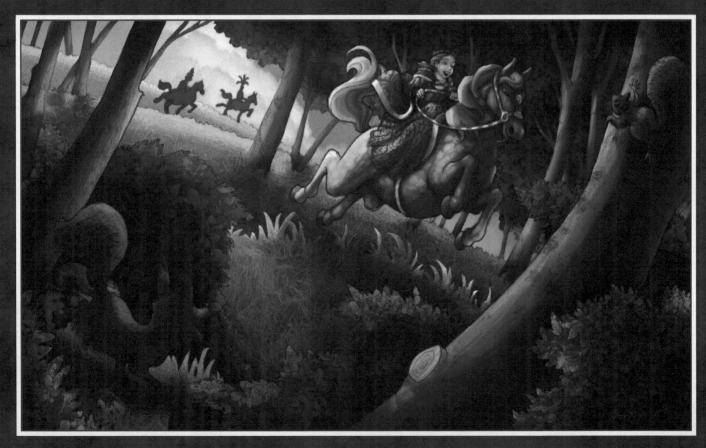

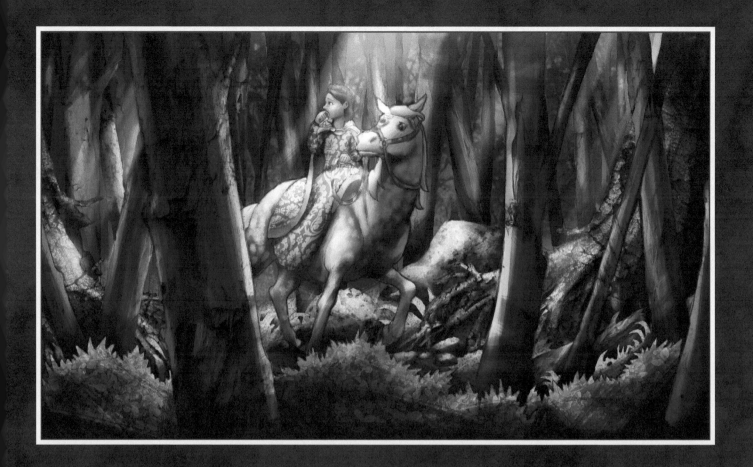

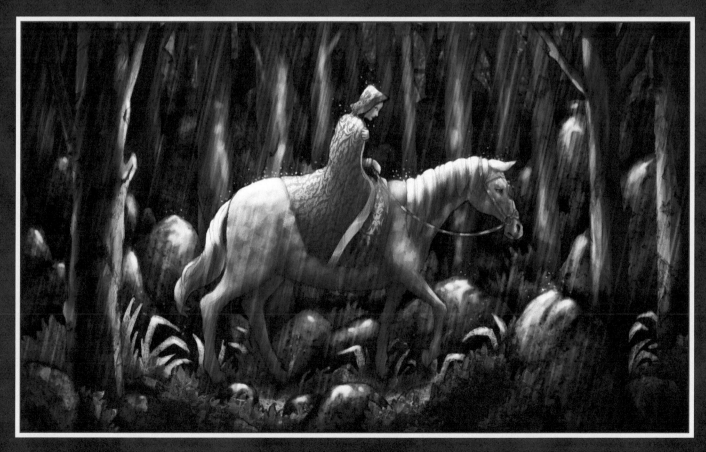

"A princess indeed," muttered the queen. "She's likely no more real than the others. Well, we shall find out!"

"We'll make you a bed, dear. Do stay through the storm!" insisted the queen.

"Hello," said the prince.

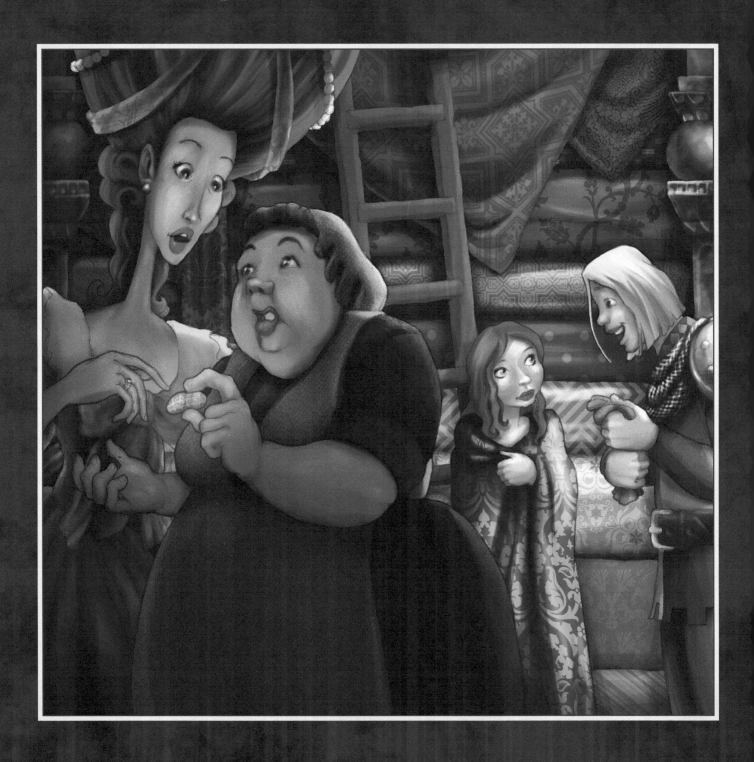

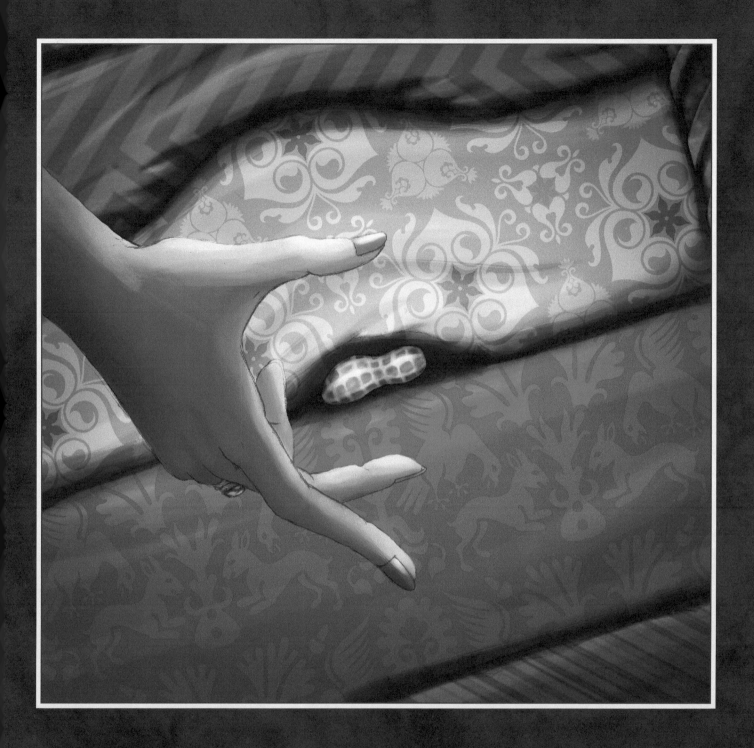

"We haven't any peas," whispered the maid. "I hope this'll do!"

"Good enough!" said the queen, slipping the peanut between two mattresses.

"Sleep well," said the queen with a wink to the maid.

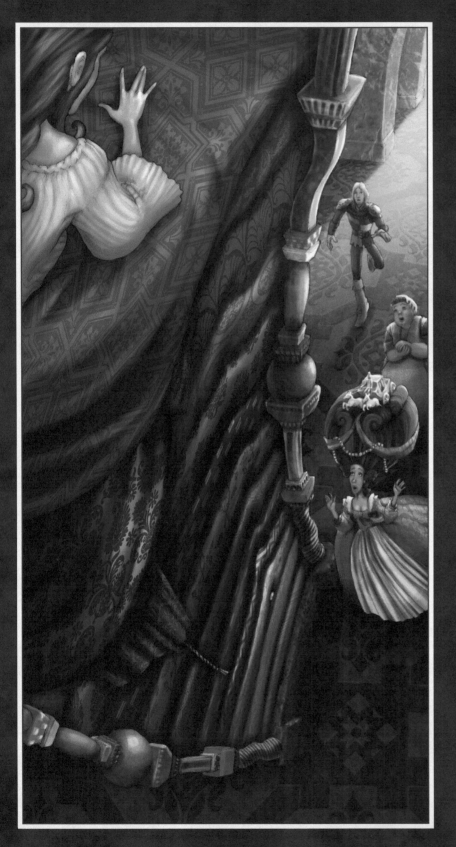

But before you could say peanut

brittle...

the queen was summoned.

"It's the princess!" cried the maid. "She's rather unwell!"

"Unwell indeed!" exclaimed the queen.

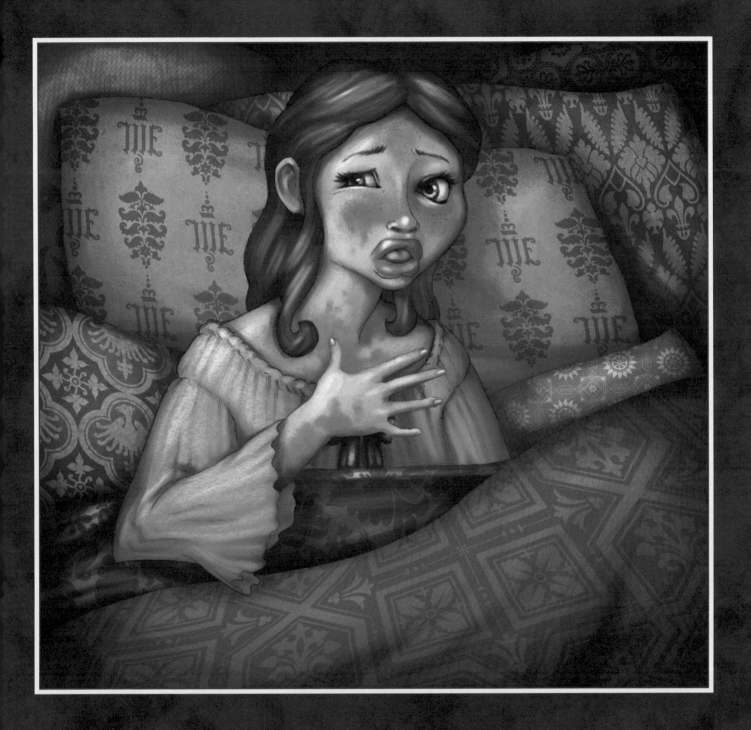

"She has more hives than the village bee farm," said the maid.

"And her tongue," gasped the queen. "It's wider than the castle moat!"

"Worry not," soothed the prince, "the doctor's on the way."

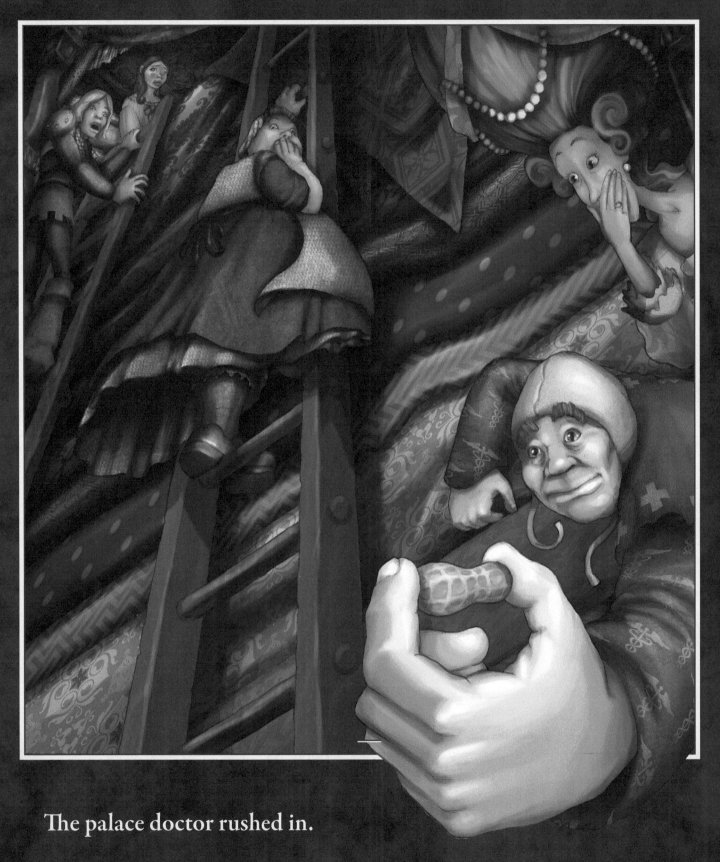

The palace doctor rushed in.

"Aha!" he said, spotting the peanut.

"She is a real princess!" exclaimed the queen.

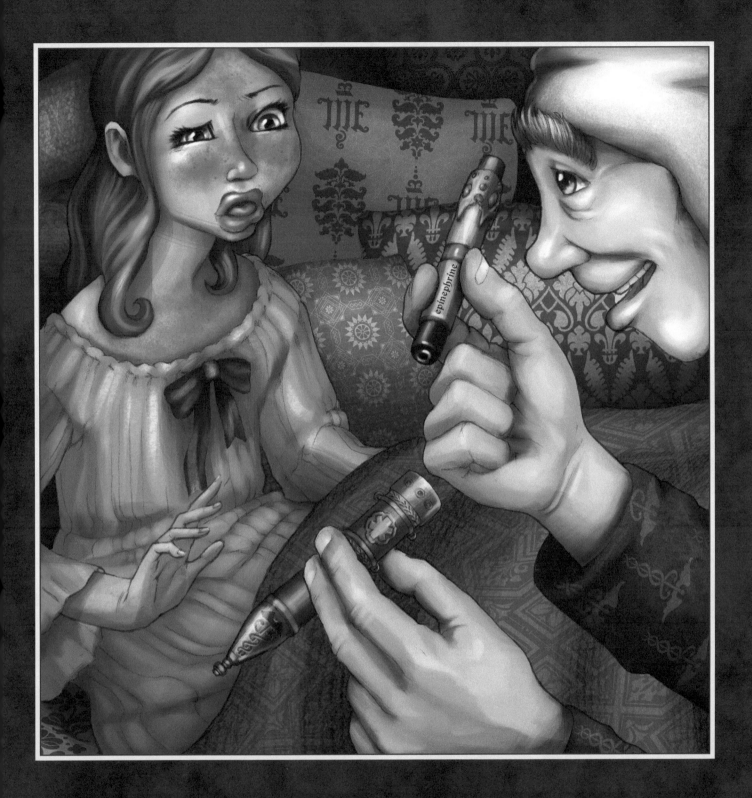

"Is that a little sword?" said the prince. "Are you preparing to fight a tiny dragon?"

"Epinephrine injection," said the doctor.

Then through her gown, into her thigh, it went.

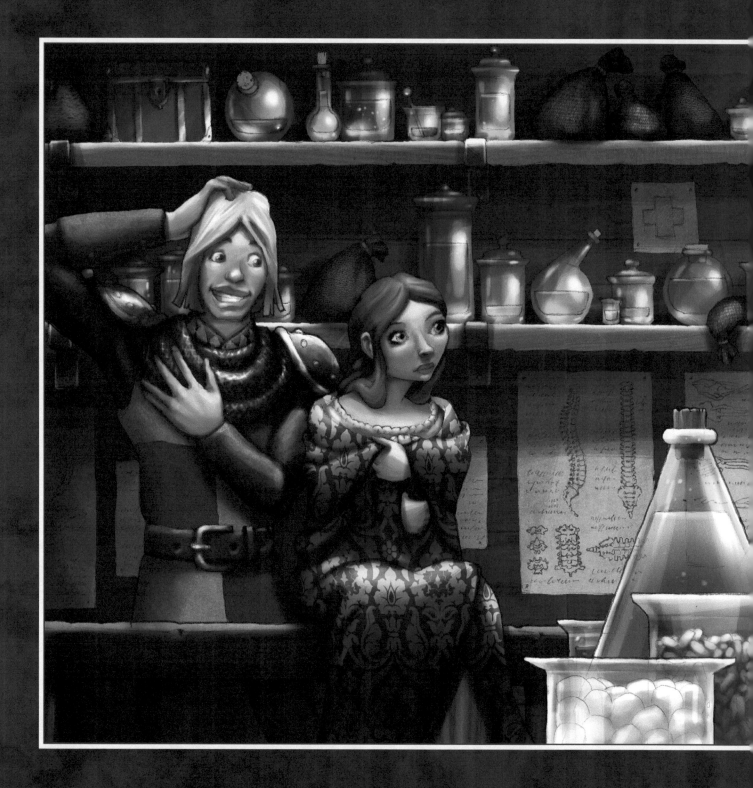

Soon she was breathing with ease.

"My heart's beating fast," said the princess. "Mine too," said the prince.

They rushed her to the royal hospital to keep a close eye on her.

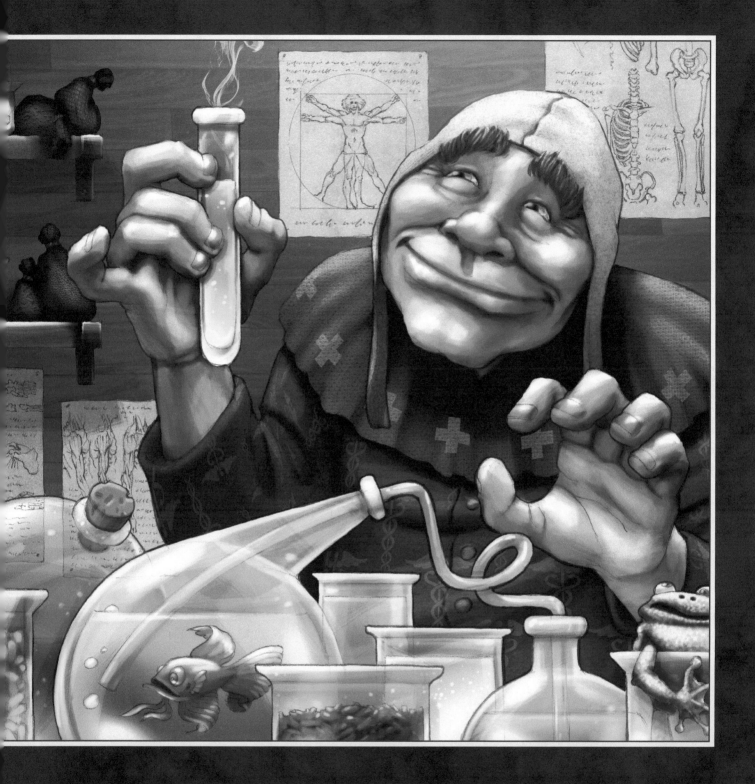

"Allergies," said the doctor, "they can come and go at any age."

"This antihistamine will help," he said, "and you may need another injection."

"If it makes me feel better," said the princess bravely.

Later she had a blood test, and a skin test for other allergies.

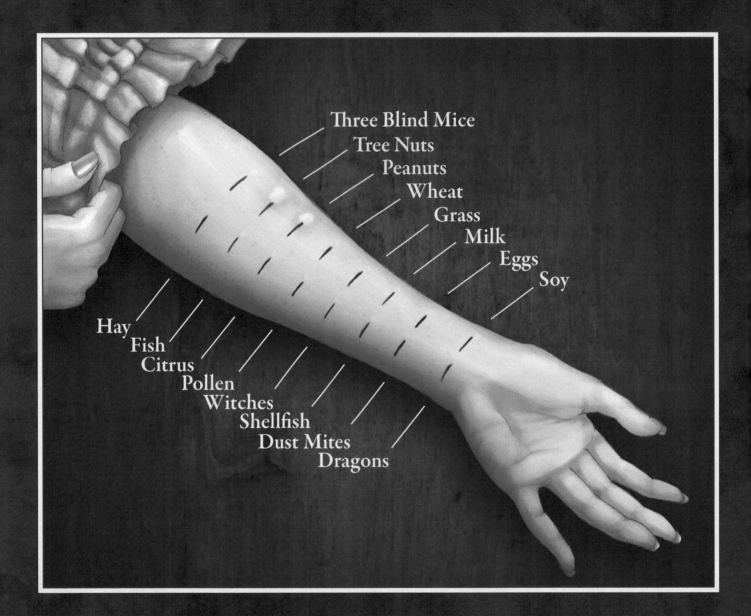

Three Blind Mice
Tree Nuts
Peanuts
Wheat
Grass
Milk
Eggs
Soy

Hay
Fish
Citrus
Pollen
Witches
Shellfish
Dust Mites
Dragons

"No peanuts, no tree nuts," said the doctor, "for any of you in the castle."

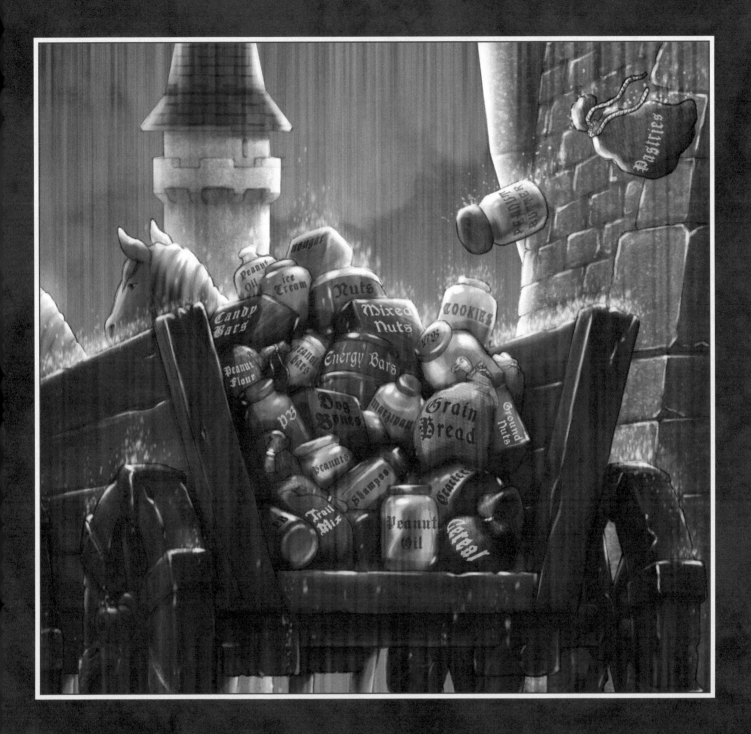

He gave the queen a list of foods that might have nuts.

"Oh my!" exclaimed the queen. "Check every label in the castle!
Leave no food unturned," she decreed. And, the clearing out began.

The prince's favorite snack, peanut butter, was the first to go.

They made the princess a comfortable new bed. No peanuts. No peas.

She stayed a fortnight, while the storm kept on.

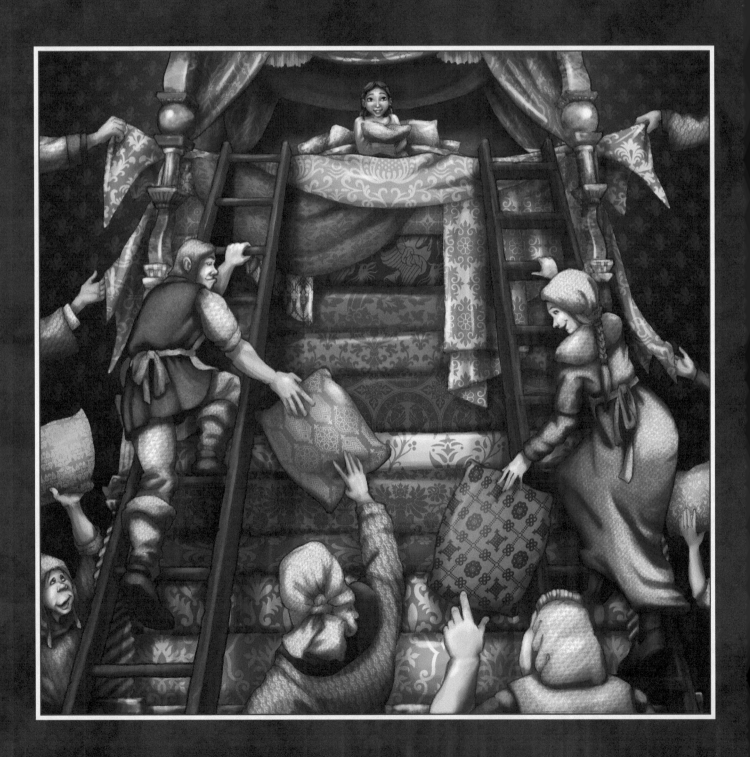

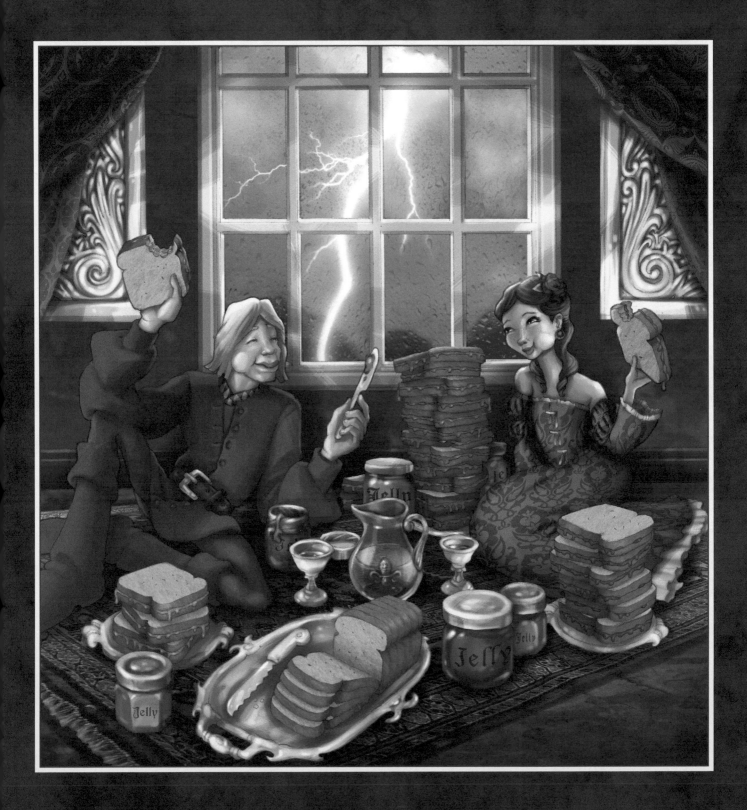

The prince was her constant companion.

But this change in eating, and having to wash hands after every new guest, was all so much for the princess.

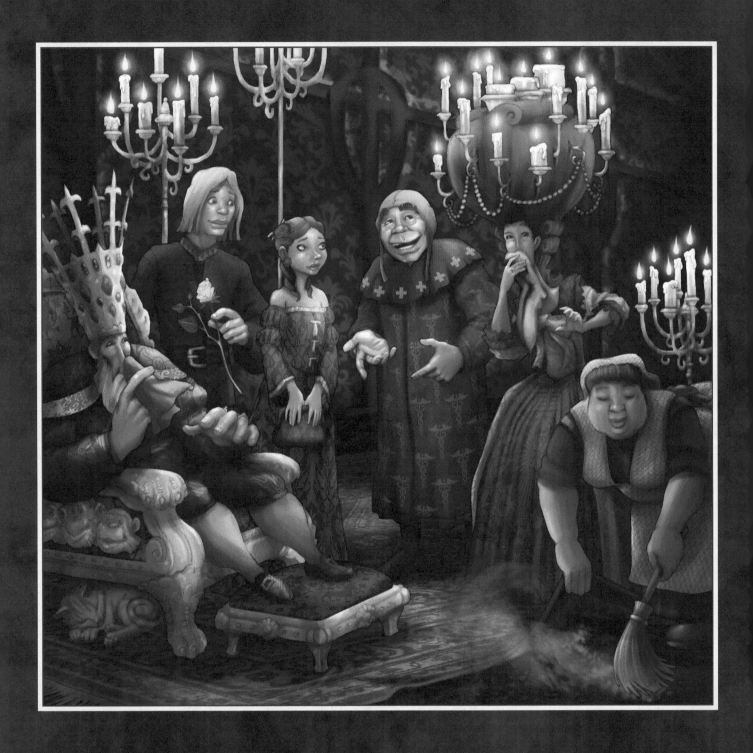

"Why me?" she asked the doctor.

"Ahh, but princesses are extraordinary, and extraordinary people have great sensitivities."

"It's true! I'm allergic to cats," proclaimed the king.

"I'm allergic to dust," sniffled the queen, eyeing the maid.

"And I'm allergic to living without my real princess," said the prince. "I shall give up peanut butter sandwiches forever if I may have your hand!"

"Oh, yes! You may have my hand...that is, if you haven't had any peanut butter today!?" said the princess, smiling.

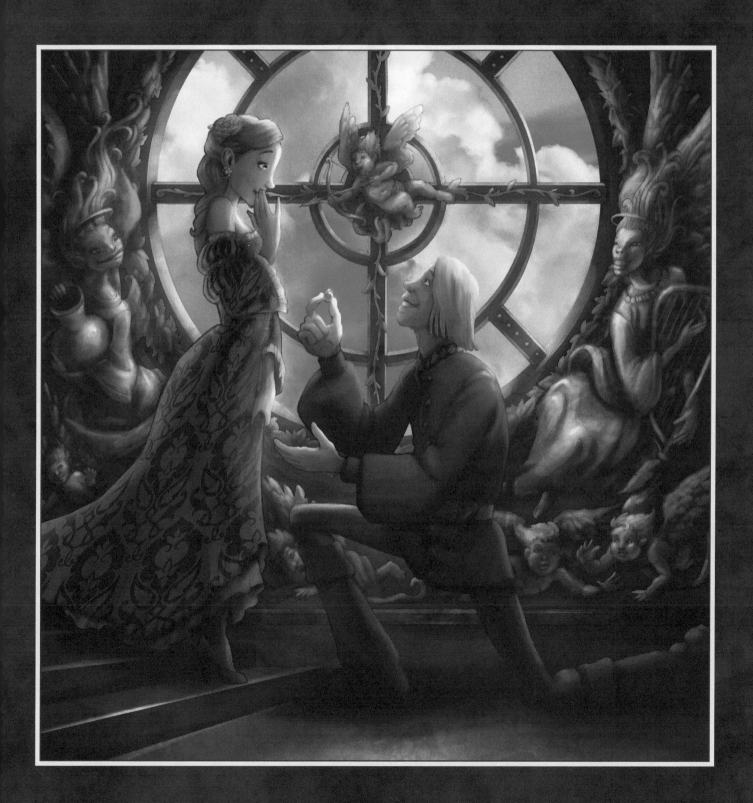

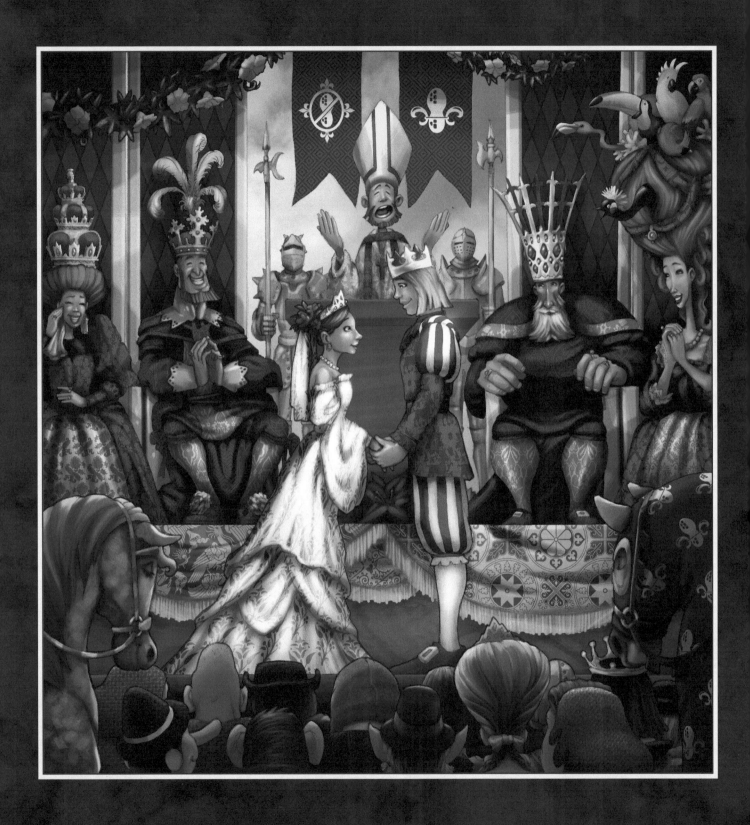

And soon they were wed, and lived their days happily, in a peanut and tree nut–free castle.

Well, almost nut–free!

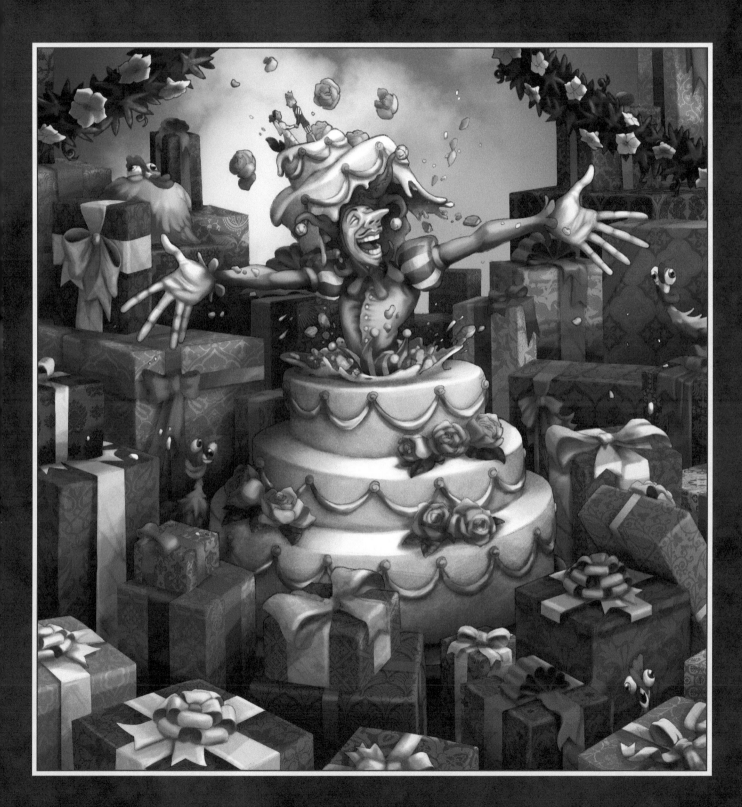

Illuminating Food Allergies: A Guide for Castle Scholars

What is a food allergy? Food allergy occurs when the immune system mistakenly attacks a food protein. Ingestion of the offending food may trigger the sudden release of chemicals, including histamine, resulting in symptoms of an allergic reaction. The symptoms may be mild (rashes, hives, itching, swelling, etc.) or severe (trouble breathing, wheezing, loss of consciousness, etc.). One in 17 children age 3 and under has a food allergy.

What are the common symptoms of a reaction? Symptoms may include one or more of the following: a tingling sensation in the mouth, swelling of the tongue and the throat, difficulty breathing, hives, vomiting, abdominal cramps, diarrhea, drop in blood pressure, and loss of consciousness. Symptoms typically appear within minutes to two hours after the person has eaten the food to which he or she is allergic.

What is the best treatment for food allergy? Strict avoidance of the allergy-causing food is the only way to avoid a reaction. Reading ingredient labels for all foods is the key to avoiding a reaction. If a product doesn't have a label, individuals with a food allergy should not eat that food. If you have any doubt whether a food is safe, call the manufacturer.

Is there a cure for food allergies? Currently, there are no medications that cure food allergies. Strict avoidance is the only way to prevent a reaction. Many people outgrow their food allergies.

What is the best treatment for a food allergy reaction? Epinephrine, also called adrenaline, is the medication of choice for controlling a severe reaction. It is available by prescription as a self-injectable. If someone has been prescribed this medication, they should carry it with them at all times!

What is the difference between a skin prick test and a blood test for allergy? A skin prick test or a blood test are designed to measure a protein called IgE that is involved in many types of food allergic reactions. A skin prick test is usually less expensive and can be done in the doctor's office. The doctor places a drop of the substance being tested on the patient's forearm or back and pricks the skin with a probe, allowing a tiny amount to enter the skin. If the patient is possibly allergic to the substance, a wheal (mosquito bite-like bump) will form at the site within about 15 minutes. The test is only slightly uncomfortable, generally not painful, and there is no bleeding. The blood test is sent to a medical laboratory, where tests are done with specific foods to determine whether the patient has IgE antibodies to that food. The results are usually received within one week.

What are some high risk foods for people with peanut/tree nut allergies? Cookies, baked goods, candy, ice cream, frozen yogurts, marzipan, nougat, Asian, African, and other ethnic dishes, cereals, chili, spaghetti sauce, chocolate, crackers, egg rolls, hydrolyzed plant and vegetable protein, peanut oil, peanut flour, peanut butter, other nut butters, and artificial nuts.

* Note: Most information above provided by the Food Allergy and Anaphylaxis Network (FAAN). Please visit their site for more information at: www.foodallergy.org

Allergy Definitions: For One and All!

Allergic Reaction – If you have an allergy, your body will have a reaction. Some reactions are: itchiness, watery eyes, runny nose, coughing, wheezing, rash, hives, a tingly feeling in (or around) your mouth, feeling tired or weak, feeling sick, stomach cramps, throwing up, part or all of your face getting puffy. You might get croaky, or lose your voice, or have trouble breathing.

Allergist – This is a doctor who has special training to figure out if someone has allergies. The "allergist" decides how to treat the person.

Allergy – When a person gets sick from something that should be harmless, it is called an "allergy." It can come from eating a food like peanuts. Or from swallowing something, like a medicine, called penicillin. It can be breathed in, like pollen from plants. It may get onto the skin, like poison oak or ivy. Or, it may get under the skin, like a bee sting.

Anaphylaxis – This is when a person has a very big (severe) allergic reaction. They might get hives. Their body parts might get swollen (like their throat or tongue). It might be hard to talk or breathe. The person could feel dizzy too, and they may faint. When someone has this, they need a medicine called epinephrine right away, and they might need to hurry to a hospital.

Antihistamine – This is a kind of medicine. It helps someone with an allergy feel better.

Epinephrine (Injector) – This is a medicine that goes into the skin (like a really fast shot). It helps someone who has an allergic reaction called "anaphylaxis."

Food Allergies – Some allergies come from food. Foods that some people are allergic to are: milk, eggs, peanuts, tree nuts, fish, shellfish, soy, and wheat. There are other foods that can also cause allergies.

Hives – Bumpy, itchy skin that happens because of an allergy.

Immune System – This is what your body uses to fight off the things that are bad for it, like the flu. The body sends out chemicals that attack the body's enemies. Sometimes, like with allergies, the body is confused and attacks things that are not bad for it.

Peanuts – These are not actually nuts, but are from the family of legumes. Other legumes are beans and peas. They grow from the ground.

Prick Test/Blood Test – These are two different ways for a doctor to check if someone has allergies. A "prick test" is when teeny tiny amounts of allergens (things that people might be allergic to) are put onto the skin for a few minutes so the doctor can see if the skin gets red bumps that might feel itchy. With a "blood test," a laboratory checks a small amount of someone's blood for signs of allergies.

Tree Nuts – These nuts are a type of dry fruit that grow on trees and do not split apart when they are ripe. Most nuts are tree nuts.

CPSIA information can be obtained
at www.ICGtesting.com
Printed in the USA
BVHW022255230921
617324BV00002B/49